IN
RUDE
HEALTH

The Funniest and Most Explicit

Stories from the NHS

First published October 2013

Freight Books
49-53 Virginia Street
Glasgow, G1 1TS
www.freightbooks.co.uk

ISBN 978-1-908754-33-2
eISBN 978-1-908754-34-9

Printed and bound by Bell and Bain, Glasgow

Introduction

We are sick. We are dirty, kinky and sexually dysfunctional. We commit stupid acts in the heat of the moment, play with tools we don't know how to use, and generally hurt ourselves – a lot. And when we aren't suffering from some awful internet-trawled illness we are totally convinced that we are. Luckily for us, we have the National Health Service on hand to pick up the pieces.

The NHS is a beautiful thing. A free healthcare system, visible proof that we live in a society that looks after its citizens. A health service where you can get treated for whatever you want whenever you need it, day or night. Be it an eel up the arse, or an urgent case of blue legs, our highly-trained health professionals are on call.

This book is full of the very best stories gleaned from those at the frontline, a collection of the weirdest accidents and patients they have attended, the ones that keep them smiling through a seventeen hour shift, or at least get them in to work the next day. A&E is a common spawning ground for these outlandish tales but the net was cast wider, to dentists, GPs, ambulance drivers, midwives, call handlers, first responders and the like.

As one would expect, all stories are supplied anonymously – to protect the innocent as well as the guilty. I'm hugely grateful to all those NHS workers who gave me material, tales that made me both laugh out loud and sometimes weep with despair… But, most of all, hearty thanks go to the Great British Public, whose imagination and inventiveness in finding methods to put itself in harm's way knows no bounds. For your perversion, stupidity and ignorance – I salute you.

Robbie Guillory

Cat and Mouse

An unconscious 30-year-old man was brought in to us by ambulance. His girlfriend had found him lying naked on the floor of his bathroom and called 999. Upon examination, he was found to have a large lump on his forehead and, strangely, several scratches on his scrotum. The lump was obviously from a fall of some kind, but we couldn't work out the cause of the scratches until he'd woken up.

He said he had been cleaning his bathtub while naked, kneeling on the floor beside the tub. His cat, apparently transfixed by the rhythmic swaying of his scrotum, lunged forward, sinking its claws into this deliciously pendulous target. The man wasn't sure what had happened next, but clearly he'd jerked forward to protect his package and cracked his skull on the edge of the bath.

A&E Consultant, Milton Keynes

The Eyes Have It

A few years ago I was working nights at an inner-city A&E in Manchester. A man staggers in, clearly the worse for wear drink-wise, and tells the front desk that he can't get his contact lenses out. Apparently they would come halfway out but then always snap back in again, and were causing him agony. A nurse attempted to get them off with a suction pump but to no avail, and the patient was getting more and more panicked, so they called me in to have a look. I checked both eyes, twice, but couldn't find any sign of lenses. The man had been trying to rip out his own corneas.

Doctor, Milton Keynes

Bottoming Out

I remember a case where a man reported to his GP complaining of severe constipation, and quite considerable pain. After some persuasion he revealed that he and his boyfriend had been getting into some very risqué sex games, and recently they had had the idea of pouring plaster of Paris into his bottom using a funnel. This had hardened, unfortunately, and thus the constipation and pain. The GP referred him to our hospital, and it was my privilege to remove what turned out to be a pretty perfect cast of his rectal passage, along with - somewhat surprisingly - a squash ball.

Nurse, Cambridge

Miracle Cure

A woman came into my A&E while I was
on the front desk and the following
conversation took place:

'What's the problem?'

'I've got appendicitis!'

'What makes you say it is appendicitis?'

'Because I had it before, when I was
twelve! I had to go to hospital and have
an operation!'

'You had your appendix taken out?'

'Yes!'

'And you think you've got appendicitis?'

'Oh...'

Needless to say, it was a touch of the
shits.

Nurse, Bournemouth

Chilli Con Vagi

My colleague, a GP, recently told me about this patient he'd had. She came in to a drop-in appointment, refused to sit down in the waiting area, was sweating profusely and highly agitated, so the receptionist decided to bump her up the list a bit. When she came in she still wouldn't sit down and blurted out, 'I've got a chilli in my vagina!'

'Umm, ok, is it stuck?' my colleague asked.

'No, I just want some advice please!'

'Well, my advice would be that you take the chilli out of your vagina, and never put it back in again. Not only is it dangerous, they are far better used in a good curry.'

'Thank you!'

'Would you like to talk about *why* you've got a chilli in your vagina?'

'No thanks, you've been a lot of help already,' she said, and was out the door before the GP could say another word.

Doctor, Norwich

Speed Dogging

A story was doing the rounds in my area recently about a teenager with ADHD who had been taking dexamphetamine with some friends (the drug was prescribed by his local community Adolescent Psychiatry service to stop him setting fire to his homework, among other things...). His parents had brought him in when they found him in their attic in a very, shall we say, incoherent state. Once he'd come off his high somewhat, the doctor wanted to ask him if he's been doing anything that might put him at risk of contracting AIDS. The boy thought for a while and then said, '...screwing the dog?'

Doctor, Truro

Funny Games

A man had inserted an acupuncture needle in his penis. We found this out only after having X-rayed, following complaints of a severe pain in his stomach. It had reached his bladder. When we showed him this X-ray, he admitted having put it there, 'for fun'.

Nurse, Leicester

Buried Treasure

I have personally removed the following
items of flotsam and jetsam from various
rectums over the past forty years:
  Several shapes of bottle
  Sex toys galore
  One aubergine
  A snapped broomstick handle
  The handle of an axe, with the axe head
  attached but not inserted
  The bauble from the end of a curtain rod
  (became unscrewed, apparently)
  A light bulb (unbroken, thankfully)
  One fluorescent tube
  A champagne glass (it had smashed)
  A full jar of instant coffee
  A prosthetic arm
  A plethora of toothbrushes
  Only one cucumber, oddly
  A marble pestle (luckily no mortar)
  A large rubber 'Hulk' fist (and again,
  two years later)
  Many eggs
  A can of Carnation condensed milk

Limes
A mobile phone, curiously not set to
vibrate mode
A stapler.

Surgeon, Bristol

Beardbugs

I was once assisting a dentist as she was doing a filling. The patient was a bear of a man, with an imposing beard. Suddenly, as I was reaching for a packing pad, I noticed an ant running across the tray where we kept the tools. Not wanting to cause undue alarm, I decided to ignore it, and swapped the tools for sterile ones. Once the patient left I asked the dentist if he'd seen any ants, thinking we might have a pest problem, to which she replied, 'It was the patient. His beard was seething with them, but I didn't want to upset him by mentioning it. They kept trying to climb up my gloves.'

Dental assistant, Newcastle

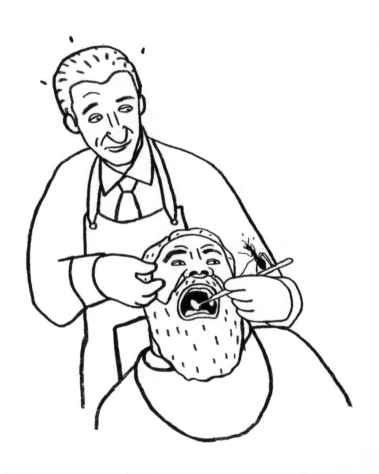

Premium Call Rate

This incident was related to me by a
senior colleague who worked in the days
when general practitioners still did lots
of routine house calls and when doors were
never locked. He knocked on the door of
a female patient who called for him to
walk straight in. He did so, to find her
lying naked in a tin bath in front of the
fire. She looked up and said cheerfully,
'Oh it's you, doctor! I thought it was the
insurance man.'

Doctor, Ayrshire

Currant Affairs

During our anatomy years, a group of us had to dissect the green body of an elderly female with a proud risus sardonicus (a death-mask grin).

As the dissection progressed to the lower extremities, our tutor decided to demonstrate how a PV (a treatment applied to the vagina) would have to be done later in clinical training. As he withdrew his gloved middle finger, sitting happily on the tip of it was a raisin. He mused in wonderment, 'How did that get there?' A mutter response came from our worldly-wise colleague, having partied well the night before:

'Maybe she had a bun in the oven!'

Surgeon, Brighton

Turd Time Lucky

A young GP Registrar, who cut her teeth on squelchy carpet home visits in urban Ayrshire, later moved to a greater calling in deepest Drumchapel, Glasgow. Early one afternoon, summoned to minister to a sick child, she found herself walking up a nominal garden path, through the standard avenue of discarded couches, mattresses and old cookers to the battle-scarred door of a tenement, outside of which sat a big dog.

Receiving the customary no answer to her knock, she called out 'Doctor here!' and as she slowly opened the door, the big dog immediately bounded upstairs ahead of her. She followed it cautiously into a dimly-lit living room, where half a dozen assorted, multi-pierced male and female slackers sat menacingly around the walls in a fug of wacky baccy, watching her intently.

Uncomfortable and self-conscious – and from past experience unwilling to kneel on the floor – she crouched beside the settee to examine the florid chickenpox of her young patient. As she did so, she was conscious, out of the corner of her eye, of the big dog arching its back in the middle of the room and dumping a huge turd on the threadbare carpet.

Nobody moved. Not a word was said. Appalled by this lumpen display of total indifference to filth, she hurriedly scribbled a script for Calpol and Calamine Lotion, handed it to the mother, and beat a hasty retreat towards fresh air and civilisation. Nobody moved.

As she exited the room and closed the door in relief, behind her she heard someone cry:

'Haw, Doctor! Yev forgotten yer fuckin dug!'

Doctor, Glasgow

Not Getting Through

A 92-year-old woman had a full cardiac arrest at home and was rushed to the hospital. After about thirty minutes of unsuccessful resuscitation attempts, the old lady was pronounced dead. The doctor went to tell the lady's 78-year-old daughter that her mother didn't make it. 'Didn't make it? Where could they be? She left in the ambulance forty-five minutes ago!'

Doctor, Sunderland

Stuck in the Middle of You

We were on call in our ambulance, when an ESA (Embarrassing Sexual Accident) came on the screen. The notes said that a couple had got stuck while in the midst of coital passion, with the man unable to remove his member. The notes went on to say that 'The female is not in pain, but the male is feeling the pinch.' This was enough to have us laughing uncontrollably; but what was more, the caller's name had been recorded as 'Male – friend on scene'. Sadly he had scarpered by the time we arrived.

Ambulance driver, London

Fire in the Hole

'In retrospect, lighting the match was my big mistake, but I was only trying to retrieve the hamster,' Philip told colleagues in the Severe Burns Unit he'd been rushed to.

Philip and his partner William had been admitted for emergency treatment after a felching session had gone seriously wrong. 'I pushed a cardboard tube up his rectum and slipped Gerald, our Campbell's hamster, in,' he said. 'As usual, Will shouted, "Apocalypse!" – our safe word that he'd had enough. I tried to retrieve Gerald, but he wouldn't come out again, so I peered into the tube and struck a match, thinking the light might attract him.'

The match must have ignited a pocket of intestinal gas and a flame shot out of the tube, igniting Philip's hair and severely burning his face. It also set fire to Gerald's fur and whiskers, which in turn ignited a larger pocket of gas further up the intestinal tract, propelling the hamster out like a cannonball.

Philip suffered second-degree burns and a suspected broken nose from the impact of the hamster, while William suffered first and second-degree burns to his anus and lower intestinal tract.

I never heard what happened to Gerald the hamster.

GP, Wolverhampton

Taking the Plunge(R)

The oddest thing that has happened in my career so far has to be the woman who Superglued a plunger to her vagina. Apparently she'd been having fun with her girlfriend when the harness for their strap-on broke. In the heat of the moment (she told us she 'wasn't thinking straight'), she thought that the plunger under the sink would give the right amount of, well, movement. After a quick wash under the hot tap (so considerate), she then tried to work out how to attach it. To cut a long story short, the pair decided in the heat of their ardour to use Superglue to affix the device. A foolish thing to do, and one that is very hard to hide whether you are sitting, lying or standing in the waiting room of A&E.

Nurse, Manchester

Foiled Again

As a pharmacist, I am often a patient's source of information about their medication. When one woman came to the pharmacy to get a refill on her suppositories, she asked me if I had any suggestions she could take to her doctor. She said that the suppositories were not working. 'And not only don't they work, they *hurt!* Sometimes they even make me *bleed*!'

I looked at her prescription, pulled some suppositories from the shelf, and opened the box for her. She then showed me that the corners of the hard foil wrapper were sharp. I cringed when I realised that she was not removing the packaging before inserting them.

Pharmacist, Croydon

Well Fly

When I was still training to be a dental assistant, this happened during one of my last practical exams. A very important exam was being graded by an observer supplemented with input from the dentist. The dentist was working on an amalgam for a filling, and I was handing him the instruments and materials as he needed them, without him having to ask. I was sweating buckets, I was so nervous. Then out of nowhere a bluebottle spirals down, and where does it land but on the tip of the patient's tongue, seemingly stone dead, on its back, no wing twitching, nothing.

Now, I can't afford to make a mistake, and I'm so nervous that all I can think is, 'What's the proper instrument for removing a dead stuck fly from a person's tongue?' I had to think fast, so I look at my tray, grabbed an amalgam carrier, and pressed it into the hands of the dentist. The dentist, a terrifying professor known for his brutal marking, grunts, takes the carrier, scoops the bug up with the large end and hands it back to me, saying, 'That was correct.'

I couldn't believe it.

Dental assistant, Warrington

Weighty Pronouncement

A couple of years ago one of my fellow midwives was an extremely large woman called Lucy, who was so large it made you want to give up eating for her. Not only was she fat, she also had a 'big personality', and with that came a very blunt way of speaking. Now, usually this wasn't a problem, as not many people argue back to someone who looks like they would happily snack on them if given the chance, but there was one incident that will always stick in my mind.

It was once considered good practice to weigh expectant mothers every time they came in for a check-up and Lucy was always one to make comment on this. So an expectant mother comes in, looking quite normal, and Lucy takes her into a cubicle. They can only have been in there for a few minutes when we hear an almighty SLAP! and the mother-to-be shouting, 'If I need to watch my weight, then we'd better send out a bloody search party for whoever is watching yours!'

   With this the mum-to-be storms out.
Thirty seconds later, Lucy emerges and
says quite calmly, 'Who's next, please?'
No one mentioned the perfect handprint in
scarlet across her right cheek.

Midwife, Padstow

A Good Lay

Last month I attended the most memorable 'accident' of my career. It was on a rare quiet night in A&E, when in waddles a man in his mid-thirties. I ask him the matter – though I can smell the booze a mile off – and he says it's his birthday, and he's been playing a drinking game. Now, whenever we hear the words 'drinking game' uttered by someone in A&E we know it isn't going to be pretty. It turned out that the final forfeit was the insertion of a carton of six eggs up the arse, and this poor sod had lost, and was now overcome with worry that they might smash inside him before he could lay them to rest, as it were. We got them out all right, and presented them back to him in an egg box to take home. Things like that that make A&E worth it.

A&E Consultant, Edinburgh

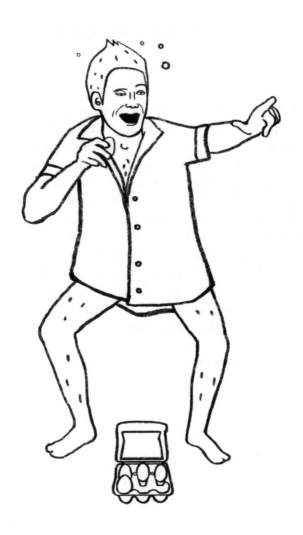

Seed Potato

I never thought this was even possible until I saw it with my own eyes. A woman came into my GP surgery complaining that there were vines growing out of her vagina. I examined her, and she certainly wasn't wrong – there was a stalk of about six inches protruding from it. Further examination revealed a potato, which was the source of the problem (sprouting as they do in warm, moist and dark environments). We never did find out just why it had been put in there, and for how long it had… germinated.

Doctor, Essex

Concrete Thinking

A fool came clumping in with one foot in a bucket. It turned out he was a self-proclaimed 'artist', and for his art he'd decided that he would like to make a cast of said foot. So he'd got a square plastic bucket, filled it with concrete, and plopped his foot straight in, sitting down in a chair, waiting for the concrete to harden enough for the cast to be made. He watched telly for several hours, ate some snacks and then, bored, worked his way through a half bottle of whisky. Waking more than half a day later, the penny finally dropped that he wouldn't have any way to get his foot out of the cement, which was now almost completely hard.

We had to anaesthetise him and then get the bloody fire brigade to break the cement off; and let me tell you, the force needed to break cement is more than enough to break bones. The post-op x-ray was quite something to behold.

Orthopaedic Surgeon, London

Full of Beans

A woman brings in her two-year-old grandson, completely distraught, and tells us that she was getting ready to give him a bath when she noticed that 'his belly button was falling off!' Now, this seemed like quite the emergency, but in fact the boy had a baked bean stuffed in his belly button.

Nurse, Birkenhead

Stuck on Repeat

A man was brought in with a bad case of concussion, which had resulted in extreme short-term memory loss. I'd walk into the room and tell him he had a concussion and he'd explain he had one when he was a kid. This was repeated every time I walked into the room. After about 10 times of doing this, I walked in and told him he had a concussion and he'd had one before when he was a kid.

Mind blown. Priceless.

Consultant neurologist, Glasgow

Frank Exchange

Me: Hello, my name is Frank and I'm the duty doctor tonight.

Patient: Hi Frank, I'm a junkie and I'm off my fucking head.

It doesn't get much better than that.

A&E Registrar, Brighton

Love Buzz

We had a young lady in recently with a trapped foreign body. A sex toy, it turns out. This little exchange occurred during examination:

Patient: Can you feel where it is?

Me: Yes.

Patient: Can you pull it out?

Me: I don't think so; we'll have to take you into theatre, I'm afraid.

Patient: Before we go there, any chance you can please SWITCH IT OFF!

Obstetrics & Gynaecology Registrar, London

Rash Behaviour

A woman came into A&E worried because her legs had taken on a bluish tinge. Upon examination it was a case of newjeansitis.

Doctor, Swansea

Early Bird

At 8am one morning, a man rushes into our surgery, carrying a small Tupperware box. He comes up to me at the counter and says, 'I've just passed a worm – it was floating in the loo after I went this morning. Here, I captured it and brought it with me.'

He smacks the box down on the countertop. It is filled with slightly off-coloured water, and there is a stringy black thing floating about in it. I'm about to get him signed in, but something about the 'worm' makes me look closer. It was a hairband.

Receptionist, Newcastle

Just Say No

So a patient was admitted to A&E on a stretcher following an overdose of painkillers after being dumped by his partner. After he had been stabilised, I was called to assess his mental state. I asked if he had taken anything else other than painkillers.

He replied 'Yes, cannabis and cocaine, but I DON'T DO HARD DRUGS!!' I love humanity.

Psychiatry Registrar, London

Running Gag

Man comes in with a bad case of gastroenteritis, and by bad I mean *terrible* – he was leaking profusely from his arse, dehydrated, in incipient circulatory shock and a state of near-constant retching. In the process of securing the diagnosis, I asked him if he'd been travelling overseas recently or eaten anything off or odd. This is what he told me:

'Well, I was at a brothel last night and I may have swallowed some water in the communal spa they have there, would that count?'

And I had to treat this guy.

Doctor, Edinburgh

Fowl Play

I'm working one of my first A&E shifts after qualifying. A distraught father runs in, carrying a small boy who has a red towel wrapped around his hand, and shouts, 'My son's been bitten by a dog!'

Naturally, we rush his son through, thinking we're in traumatic amputation territory.

In the cubicle, I gently unwrap the towel but can't see any blood or dampness – in fact, there was only the tiniest of scratches on a finger. You'd almost need a magnifying glass to see it. I ask him what happened, and this boy, who must have been only about five years old, tells me that he was bitten by a DUCK.

Nurse, Colchester

Coming Up Slowly

One of my patients comes to see me complaining of a headache from taking ecstasy. This seems pretty alarming, so I'm immediately accessing her notes with the thought to send her straight to hospital. As I'm typing, I ask when the ecstasy was taken. 'I took a pill about two years ago,' she replies. My typing slows. I ask if she's had a headache since that fateful day, to which she says, 'No, it comes and goes. I've noticed that if I've been drinking I get it really badly the next day.' I stop typing, count to ten, and gently begin to explain to her about hangovers…

GP, Aberdeen

Stained Reputation

I remember a man coming into A&E for a sore throat, and once he'd waited for three hours and I'd got him in a cubicle, he pulled out some crusty ladies' underwear and asked me if I could check some stains for DNA, as he thought his girlfriend may have been cheating.

Registrar, Bath

Dying for a Ciggy

Overheard in the waiting room of an A&E Department:
  Nurse: You seriously want to go for a smoke with a collapsed lung!?
  NO, NOT TONIGHT, SUNSHINE.

Hospital Security Officer, Liverpool

Small World

We had a very drunk but lucid road trauma patient come in one Friday night, bleeding all over the place. We had a hard time examining him because he was thrashing around. He became particularly upset when my colleague began to cut off his trousers. The doctor asked him what the matter was, at which the man threw himself back on the bed, sobbing, before shouting, 'I've got a really small cock!'

We had to promise not to laugh or stare before he let us continue.

Nurse, Portsmouth

Shaving Face

Last year I treated a woman suffering from some quite nasty lateral lacerations on her buttocks. She was very reticent about how she'd come by them. They didn't require stitches, so I cleaned them up and put a dressing on; soon enough she was good to go. As she was leaving the cubicle she turned around and said, 'Can I ask your advice on something?' I agreed, saying I'd do my best.

She went on to tell me how she'd been having sex in the shower, and the cuts were from a safety razor that had been sitting on a little shelf. The trouble was, she said, she didn't know how to tell her husband. I pointed out that he'd probably noticed when she did, as there would have been quite a lot of blood. 'That's the problem,' she said, 'it wasn't him I was shagging!'

Nurse, Belfast

Shit Happens

A man comes to our surgery complaining about his bowels. Apparently his poo usually sinks, but that morning it floated, so he thinks it probably needs checking out. He's even brought us a sample in a ziplock bag. All I can do is gaze at him in shock, before asking him to take a seat.

GP, Wrexham

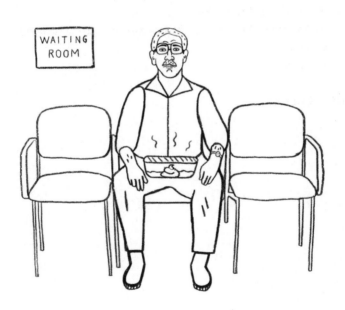

Handy

An interesting way to start a day of work:
A man comes in to my GP surgery. I ask him
what the matter is.

Patient: 'I can't stop masturbating in
public.'

OK...

GP, Cardiff

Horsing Around

A woman arrived at A&E with a nose that had been simply crushed and a pair of black eyes that would make a boxer wince. As I was treating her I asked her how it happened, and when I found her to be unwilling to talk about it, alarm bells began ringing that her injuries may have been a result of domestic abuse.

I asked her outright if her partner did this to her, to which she shook her head. I pressed her, told her not to be afraid and that we had mechanisms to help, to which she exclaimed, 'No, no, you don't understand! I haven't been punched – I was head-butted… by my horse.'

It turned out she'd be trying to move said equine's salt lick, which went down very badly and earned her a nose-to-nose jousting match.

A&E Consultant, Perth

My Body is a Temple

A woman is brought in to our A&E by the paramedics having been found collapsed by the side of the road. When the urine toxicity screen comes back, it is positive for a whole host of opiates and stimulants. After a while, she begins to come round, but when I offer her a nicotine patch (since she can't go out to smoke), she refuses, stating, 'Oh no, I don't take anything that might damage my skin!'

Nurse, London

Golden Balls

It always amazes me how much fun people have in their golden years. An elderly male came in to the surgery with a steel cock ring stuck behind his scrotum and penis, both of which were swollen to four times their usual size (he told us with pride). I asked him how long he had been in this predicament, to which he replied, 'Three days.'

I asked, 'Why didn't you come in sooner?' His answer: 'I could still pee, and the wife was happy…'

Consultant Urologist, Leicester

Killing with Kindness

Always beware a trained first aider.

A group of friends are walking along a river and come across a man lying unconscious on the river bank. Most of them get on their mobile phones and call ambulances, while one of them, the Trained First Aider, leaps into action and 'does resuscitation'. Our ambulance crew arrives to find one man sitting on the patient's belly, thumping his chest with his fist like he's trying to put a nail in, whilst another well-wisher pours water onto the poor bastard's face.

We thanked them for their efforts, naturally.

Paramedic, Bristol

X Marks the Cock

A boy, about 13 years old, and his mother came into A&E, the mother having dragged the boy in because he was complaining of nasty 'digestive' problems. He had convinced her he was fine, but eventually he couldn't hide the bleeding coming from his anus.

We took him in for X-Rays and see, clear as day, a large rubber cock, maybe 13 inches in length. The thing had wedged itself inside his bowels, was pushing on the walls of his intestine and had three days' worth of faeces piled on top of it.

I took him into a private room and asked if there is anything he wants to tell me before they discuss specifics with his mother. I said that we had found an 'object' lodged in his lower intestine and that it is going to need to be removed surgically. His response: 'Oh. I may have sat on a marker pen...'

Poor kid, just experimenting with his sexuality. With a 13" black rubber cock.

Surgeon, Oxford.

Maggot Brain

This happened a couple of years ago. Having cut my teeth in the Royal Army Medical Corps, I have been a doctor for getting on for forty years and there isn't much that makes me queasy anymore, but I have to say, this bowled me for six.

I now work as a GP and I was attending to a man, maybe in his thirties, who came to my minor surgery list with what looked like a particularly angry cyst on the top of his head. It was very distended and painful to the touch, so needed draining immediately.

I embarked on the usual drainage procedure, but I'd only gone so far as to make a small incision when I saw something was not right. There was something moving in there, visible through the small cut. I made the cut a bit bigger, and there was a huge thorny maggot, writhing about. I grabbed a tube normally used for urine samples, flicked it in and then as quickly as possible sealed it in a specimen bag, as I knew it would need to be sent to pathology. The patient and I then proceeded to throw up simultaneously.

It turned out that he had been on holiday to Central America, where he must have been bitten by a type of botfly, which laid an egg under his skin. I have never been on holiday to Central America and, now, never will.

GP, Birmingham

Lost in Space

A 21-stone woman came into A&E, complaining of a nasty yeast infection that she'd had for one month (which means it must have been quite the emergency…).

In performing a vaginal examination, I found a condom stuck quite far up, which was probably the root of the problem. To say it stank would be an understatement. After I had removed the offensive object, she asked what it was.

I told her, to which she replied, 'Oh, so that's where that went.'

Registrar, Dundee

Shit Scared

A man came in with severe abdominal pain; turned out he had such painful haemorrhoids that he'd become too scared of the pain to crap. Apparently his last defecation had been about one month previous to him coming in. One. Whole. Month.

He couldn't tolerate any of the normal treatment for chronic constipation (laxatives and enemas), so he ended up being taken to theatre where I, the most junior member of the on-call surgical team, had to claw out this monstrosity of a turd with my fingers. It was a dense mass, about 4-5 inches wide, that felt like hardened clay and smelled exactly how you might expect a ball of faecal matter that's been brewing in a dark, dank place for a month to smell.

It took a good half hour before I managed to clean him out, all while the nurses tried to stand as far away as possible and my seniors pissed themselves laughing at my various horrified expressions.

Surgeon, Belfast

Johnny Come Lately

A woman came in complaining of a 'tickle in the back of her throat' for a week, which would not go away. She'd become alarmed when a strange-coloured phlegm began to come up with each cough. I took a look in her throat and saw that there was something stuck towards the back of her nasal cavity. Also, her breath smelt like she'd been eating excrement, though she was adamant that she'd been unable to consume anything for the last couple of days. I managed to get a grip on the object with some long tweezers and began gently to pull it out - whatever it was had got really stuck to the throat lining behind the tonsils.

Turned out it was part of an edible condom, which the woman had inhaled during fellatio a fortnight previously, but she thought she'd swallowed it.

ENT Registrar, Leeds

Mythical Beast

Last Christmas, an unconscious man was admitted to our neurology ward, having sustained a head injury linked to a high blood alcohol level. We found him a bed, removed his suit, and the nurse went to insert a catheter (so he didn't wet the bed). Suddenly she gasped 'Oh my, look at this!' I went over.

Tattooed on his foreskin was a small white unicorn. Sadly, my shift ended before he could wake up, so I never got to ask him for the story behind his magical creature.

Nurse, Walsall

Miso Horny

We had a patient who had complications caused by noodles being inserted into his urethra and ending up in his bladder. The surgeon who extracted them said it was the weirdest looking ramen he'd ever seen.

Nurse, Southampton

Seeking Illumination

I like the story about the guy who
inserted a lubed-up lightbulb for sexual
kicks and, three days later, had passed
neither the lightbulb nor anything else.
So they took him into a cubicle and
made him assume the kneeling position,
introduced lots of oil and then slipped
three Foley catheters, each with a balloon
secured to the end, around the lightbulb.
They inflated the balloons and applied
gentle traction to the Foleys and waited
for about ten minutes until the anus
dilated enough to permit the passage of
the lightbulb.

And a torrent of faecal matter.

Nurse, Norwich

Please Release Me

As a student doctor, it was my duty to help file printed reports. I once came across the X-ray report of a patient with one of those telescopic umbrellas lodged in his rectum – all those moving parts were quite a sight, rather like a mechanical spider.

As I went to place it in the correct file, I couldn't help read the notes by the surgeon who removed it: it was noted that he considered it 'extremely important not to disengage the spring lock during removal.'

Doctor, Sheffield

Loose Nuts

I will never forget the man who got his penis trapped in a ring spanner. He had been masturbating with the greased-up wrench – no, I can't imagine it either – and it got stuck. His willy started to swell like crazy and after several hours he knew he had to come to A&E. We attempted to decompress the inflated member with a syringe, but that wasn't working well enough to remove it, so we were at a loss of what to do.

In the end we had to call a fireman in to get the wrench off with an industrial hacksaw. The tool (the offending wrench, not his member) was made of high-tensile steel so it took a VERY long time. And the hacksaw wasn't the most accurate of implements. We had to wear protective eyewear. The sparks were going everywhere. We had to coat his prick in cream to make sure it wasn't burned.

All the patient could say was, 'I'm sorry. I'm so, so sorry!'

Nurse, Livingston

Suck it and See

A man came into our A&E with a vacuum cleaner nozzle stuck on his penis. He had on a very long trench coat to disguise the fact. What no one could understand was why he didn't just remove the hose from the vacuum when he came in, rather than towing it behind him and his trench coat.

Nurse, Scarborough

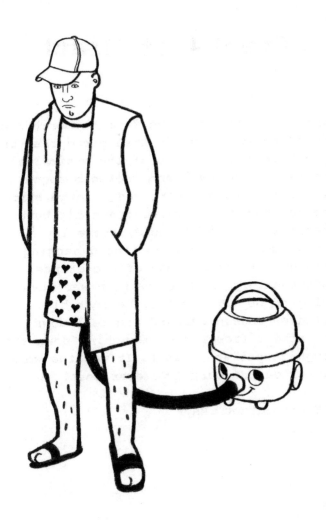

Grapes of Wrath

Some poor sod suffering from haemorrhoids wanted to see them. It transpired that he stood naked at the top of the stairs in his semi, bent over and looked between his legs, because there was a large mirror mounted there. He pulled apart his butt cheeks and, lo-and-behold, there lay the kingdom of the haemorrhoid hanging like an over-ripe bunch of red grapes. Unfortunately, such a position was never going to be very stable. He lost his balance, rocked forward and fell down the stairs face first, ploughing down the rough carpet as he went. It was the worst facial carpet burn I've ever seen.

A&E Consultant, Rhyl

Out of Puff

We once got called to attend a woman who had collapsed at her daughter's birthday party. We found her prone in the livingroom, surrounded by wailing kids and a clown in full make-up standing over her. I've never liked clowns and feared the worst.

Turned out she'd overexerted herself inflating the balloons and ended up with a pneumothorax - a collapsed lung. Saying that, I still don't like clowns.

Paramedic, Bolton

Deep Throat

A patient had been playing badminton, at some sort of championship level. Whether she was winning or not I don't know, but she seemed to have been quite a pro at it. If you've never seen a shuttlecock before, it is basically a cone made of feathers with half a polystyrene ball stuck to the pointy end, to lend weight and stop it taking someone's eye out.

Anyway, they're playing away when her opponent smashes the shuttlecock so it goes really fast, hopefully to a corner or at least out of reach. However, his aim is a bit off and the shuttlecock goes right at his opponent, and *into her mouth*.

The pointy end is at the back of her throat and making her gag, but the feathered bit of the cone is behind her teeth, because it had been hit with such force. Neither she nor the other player who hit the shot can get the shuttlecock out. Let me tell you, the sight of her sitting in the waiting room for A&E in her tennis

whites and with the most ridiculous
expression on her face... I could barely
stop myself from laughing as I cut it out.

Doctor, Walsall

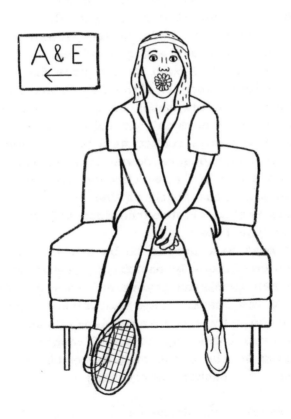

Arse-on

Bonfire night is always busy for A&E, but this incident sticks in my mind, particularly as the unfortunate patient's mates later posted the video online.

A young man had been having some fun drinking lager and throwing lit fireworks at people, when his mates suggested he 'shoot one at the moon'. He takes out a particularly large rocket he'd been saving up, pulls his trousers down, lies on his back and hooks his arms through his legs. He then slips the stand of the firework into his rectum, lights the fuse and shouts, 'Fire in the hole!'

What must have seemed to be a great idea at the time literally backfired, resulting in the man receiving severe and very painful burns to his cheeks, back and private parts.

I was told by attending friends that no one even looked up at the firework exploding as the sight of this writhing specimen was rather captivating.

Burns Specialist, Worcester

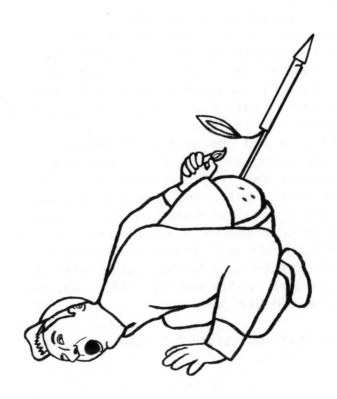

Mandible Mayhem

We can probably all remember the spitting, swearing, swivel-eyed demon that was the sports teacher at school. How he raged as we limped up and down the football pitch, surrendering goal after goal as he cursed our ineptitude and wore a groove in the turf.

Well, I had one come in to A&E who was as quiet as a mouse – completely compliant and very different to any I've experienced before or since. Of course, it could have had something to do with his injury; before he discovered this new Zen-like calm he'd been raving like the best of them at a hockey match, when he shouted so loudly and so wildly that he dislocated his jaw!

Consultant Maxillofacial Surgeon, Leeds

Rip You a New One

During the cold weather last Christmas we had to stitch up several new arse cracks. A man had cut himself when deciding to jump up and down on the roof of a bus stop, naked from the waist down, singing Jingle Bells at the top of his lungs. It had been snowing heavily for a couple of days, so when the bus stop roof shattered, there was a thick layer of snow beneath to break his fall. Sadly for him, it also meant some of the shards were stuck sharp side up, perfectly positioned to tear him a new one… or two.

Registrar, Preston

Toeing the Line

This was a first for me: a patient, who
had been chopping wood with an axe, missed
and ploughed the blade straight into his
foot (he had been wearing canvas shoes,
which had not helped at all). The stunning
thing was that he hadn't even scratched
any of the bones - just cut the skin clean
through to about halfway down the foot,
like splitting a piece of wood. Whereas
on first seeing the wound I had assumed
amputation was a distinct possibility, he
made a pretty remarkable recovery.

Reconstructive Surgeon, Cambridge

Lancing the Boil

A few years ago I remember we had a couple of young kids brought, who must have been watching too much Merlin, because they'd decided to have a jousting tournament on bicycles. They 'prepared' for this medieval folly by tying saucepans to their heads, sticking a pillow up their jumpers and using dustbin lids for shields. For lances, they use a couple of mops.

The two youngsters went to either end of the street on their bikes, and then went at each other full pelt. The results weren't pretty. The lances missed their marks, thankfully, but the bikes did not; and the two gallants were flung into each other. Teeth everywhere, huge grazes, a broken bone or two.

Charge Nurse, Nottingham

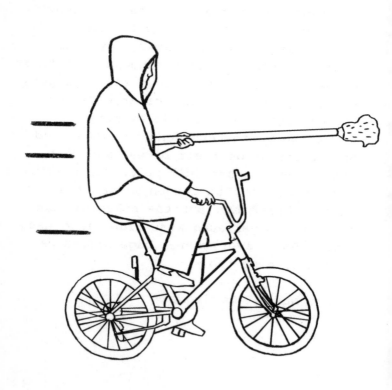

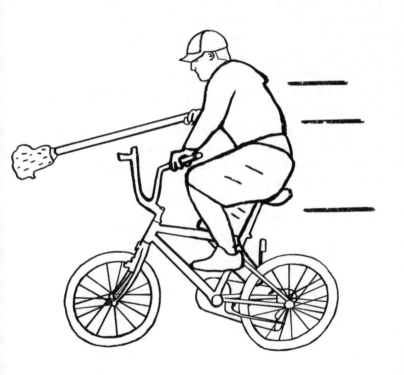

Backed Up

I had a patient who presented with a bad back, which I quickly found to be pulled back muscles. I asked if he was doing anything strenuous when the injury occurred and he went bright red and mumbled, 'Well, to be honest, I've been having quite bad constipation recently, and I think I was trying too hard to push something out.'

That's right: a man was having a shit and pulled muscles in his back. A classic case of someone needing to eat more green vegetables.

GP, Portsmouth

Nooks and Crannies

15 unusual things I've found in the crevices of incredibly fat people:
- A chicken leg
- A cheque book
- Members of the green army from the board game Risk
- A computer mouse
- Two used condoms
- A torch
- A bar of soap
- Hair scissors and a comb
- Batteries
- A ham and mustard sandwich
- A stapler
- A mousetrap
- A cricket ball
- A pocket-size Bible
- An Eagle Eyes Action Man

Community Support Nurse, Staines

Hiding to Nothing

A kinky 39-year-old guy had been copying a scene from a porn film where a live eel is put up someone's bum. Apparently he'd done it before, with complete success, but this time he lost his grip on the slippery customer, and it vanished straight into his bowels. After realising he couldn't get it out, the man rushed round to the nearest A&E, which happened to be ours...

As he came through the doors, he shouted, 'Please, please help me. An eel is moving through my body!' Naturally, he was rushed straight through, as much for his mental health as anything – and, let's face it, nobody else would have sat next to him after that.

After establishing that he was not off his head or high as a kite, our duty surgeon spent almost an hour trying to coax the eel out with a suction machine. He eventually succeeded, though the poor blighter died shortly afterwards. The eel that is. The perv was perfectly fine.

Registrar, London

Burned to be Wild

A woman was cleaning up the mess left by her hairy biker husband after he'd decided to strip his motorcycle engine on the kitchen table before putting the parts back together and taking it for a spin. One of the things he was using was a bowl of petrol (apparently it is great for getting rid of grease). She took this bowl and, not knowing what to do with the contents, decided to pour them down the loo. Her husband came back, lit a cigarette and, happy with his bike, went to the bathroom.

As he did a wee he threw his cigarette end into the loo. The explosion brought his wife running upstairs, where she found him crumpled against the wall, having been blown backwards through the door, his hair, beard, eyebrows and pubes burnt off and his clothes smouldering. She dialled 999 and we came and took care of him. Hopefully he'll remember to clean up his own mess in the future…

Paramedic, Northampton

Burst Springs

A rather large woman was brought in by ambulance with two broken legs. She'd been trampolining and had gone too high, come back down to earth and gone straight through the trampoline. Ouch.

A relative who was with her said, 'I was gardening, so I didn't see it happen, but I felt the ground shake and just instinctively knew what had happened.'

Orthopaedic Surgeon, Cardiff

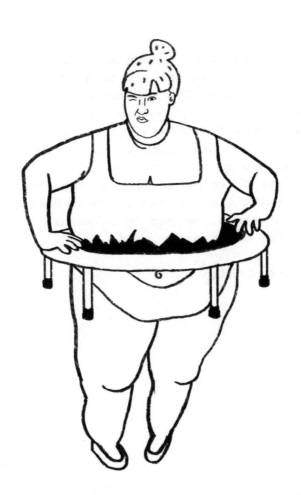

Muddy Waters

We looked after a drunken eejit who
decided to take a walk on a frozen canal
one Christmas Eve without noticing the
ice was actually just moonlight. He jumped
down from the walkway, and immediately
sank up to his waist in water, with his
legs caught in three feet of ice-cold mud.
It was three hours till he was found,
by which time he had a lovely dose of
hypothermia and had to celebrate Christmas
in the observation ward.

Nurse, Dublin

Eye on the Ball

I treated a gentleman in late middle age who had found he was having trouble peeing straight, so he decided to make some modifications to his penis. He inserted a small ball-bearing into the tip of the urethra reasoning that if it worked for a ballpoint pen, then it should improve his aim. Apparently as well as hurting like mad, and giving him a nasty urinary tract infection, it also made him into more of a sprinkler than a Deadeye Dan.

Urology Registrar, Salisbury

Patched Up

A wee old man had come to see me for a check-up, and mentioned that he'd quite like to stop smoking. Naturally I jumped on this and immediately talked to him about things that could help him achieve this. He liked the sound of patches, so I gave him a prescription for them, and then didn't see him for a few weeks. When he did eventually return, he came in slightly agitated, and explained to me that he'd been feeling very sick. I asked him to take off his top, so I could hear his chest. His whole torso was covered in patches. Apparently he hadn't read that when you put a new patch on every day, you take the old one off.

GP, Stornoway

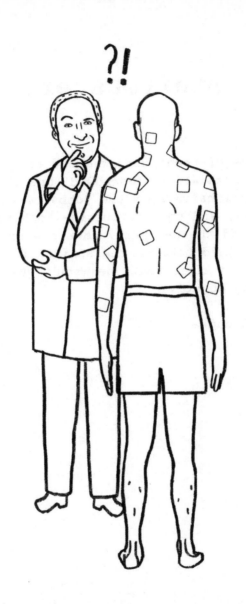

Stairmasters

A couple of teenagers, who had been in
to see a relative, 'borrowed' one of
the wheelchairs from the lobby of the
hospital, and took it outside to have a
go around the car park. Then one of them
decided he'd take on the stairs, Italian
Job-style. After that, he wasn't just
visiting anymore.

Nurse, Dundee

Come Again

Doing the pain assessment for a woman who we were pretty sure was going into labour, the following exchange took place:

Me: Is your pain intermittent or constant?

Patient: What?

Me: Does your pain come and go or is it constant?

Patient: Well, it constantly comes and goes!

Community Midwife, Poole

You Know What They Say

James was 87, the sweetest of patients, one of nature's gentlemen. One day when I was giving James a sponge bath I'd stood him up so I could wash his privates when he looked down and said, 'Have you ever seen anything so big?'

I was utterly speechless – couldn't think of anything to say.

James shook his head and said, 'My brother-in-law told me once that these have got to be the biggest bloody feet he'd ever seen!'

Geriatric Nurse, Ashford

Milking It

I'll never forget the poor woman who, when applying a homemade enema, suspected – and then, as warmth grew, suddenly realised – that, in a dimly lit room, she'd grabbed a bottle of chilli oil by mistake. There was very little we could do for her, except for filling her with milk while she lay on her front, sweating like mad and mooing with pain.

A&E Consultant, Winchester

Tap on the Head

A man was fixing his car, fiddling about under the bonnet, when he suddenly received an almighty electric shock, throwing him to the ground and giving him a nasty blow to the back of the head. He got his wife to have a look, but she couldn't see anything except a nasty graze, and so just slapped a dressing on to it. The next day, however, he started to feel really dizzy, nauseous and forgetful, so they went to the doctor's (that's me) to get it looked at. At first inspection I couldn't see anything more than his wife could, but the dizziness was a bit alarming, so I thought we'd better scan his brain to make sure there was no evolving bleed or anything like that.

I sent him into A&E and, well, what they found was remarkable. Rather than an electric shock throwing him back, what the man had received was a bullet to the back of the head. It must have been a ricochet or fired from some distance, otherwise he'd have died for sure, but there it was, a bullet lodged in his skull. They do say that Nottingham has a lot of gun crime, but I'd yet to experience anything like that.

GP, Nottingham

Fence Corrective

A man was admitted to our hospital soaking, with a sore penis and blotchy lumps all over his bald head.

Apparently he'd been driving through the countryside and needed to stop and have a pee, choosing to go in a gap in the hedge. However, strung across the gap was what turned out to be electric fencing for keeping a bull in the field behind. He got a nasty shock all the way up his cock, fainted backwards into a ditch, and got covered in nettle stings.

He admitted to me that he knew was probably okay but was worried the electric shock to his willy might have done lasting damage. My suspicion is that he thought the voltage might have turned him into some kind of superhero…

A&E Nurse, Coleraine

Ankling for Trouble

A woman appeared at our A&E and complained
that her ankle had been sore for about
three months. When I tried to find out
exactly what was wrong with it, she
insisted that I look at the other one
first - the healthy one. I insisted that
I knew exactly what a normal ankle looks
like, and that that knowledge should be
more than adequate for this examination.
At this she got furious, said that she
wanted a new nurse, and that she wouldn't
show anyone the bad ankle until they'd
seen what her normal ankle looked like.
She was waiting a long time.

Nurse, Sunderland

Rip it Up and Start Again

We were called to an attempted suicide in a student flat. A young couple had been drinking, had a fight, then made up, before falling into a deep sleep. The girlfriend had woken in the early hours, with the sensation that she was soaking wet. Turning on the bedside light and pulling back the covers, she was horrified to discover they were both drenched in blood, huge amounts of it.

She quickly worked out she was okay and it seemed her boyfriend had been driven to try and kill himself as a result of the fight the previous evening. He was unconscious. She called 999 immediately.

When we arrived she was hysterical. The bed was a mess. Like that scene in *The Godfather*. There was even blood on the walls. But something wasn't right. We couldn't find any incisions in his wrists or on his thighs. Although he was totally unconscious his pulse and breathing were normal.

After further examination, it appeared the source of the blood was around his groin area. But again no cuts. My colleague then had a brainwave. He peeled back the lad's foreskin and sure enough, his frenulum (the piece of skin that runs between the foreskin and the head of the penis - also known by Paramedics as the banjo string) was completely ripped. There was a lovely gaping wound right up to the urethra. Believe it or not, a remarkably common injury when couples have sex drunk - caused by lack of lubrication.

You have been warned.

Paramedic, Anglesey

Root of the Problem

A young lady came in to us complaining of passing blood; no pain, but the urine was red. I asked the usual questions; have you been doing anything different, strenuous or kinky – but no, she hadn't done anything unusual. I checked her vitals but couldn't find anything, so put her in a cubicle and asked for a urine sample. No blood showed up in the urine test, not even a drop – in fact, it looked like very healthy pee. We simply couldn't work it out. I asked again if she was sure she'd done nothing out of the ordinary, nothing to excess?

She thought for a moment and then the penny dropped. 'Oh yes,' she said. 'I've eating a load of beetroot this week.'

GP, Chelmsford

Pasta Joke

This tale was told to me by a man waiting in A&E in the wee hours. He'd come home from the pub and was feeling a bit peckish. He rattled through his cupboards for a little something, but all he could find was a bag of pasta (penne, from the way he was describing it). He admitted that he wasn't much of a cook, and mostly lived off microwave dinners since his wife had left. But when you're hungry, you're hungry, and in his state of inebriation decided to have a go at cooking – after all, how hard could it possibly be? So he got a pan, slapped in half a pack of butter, got it nice and hot, then chucked in the pasta and fried it up. It smelled good, but he was stirring it round and round for ages and it wasn't getting any softer, so in the end he had to eat it raw. Apparently it really hurt his gums (he insisted on showing me).

Once he'd finished his delicious supper, the beer really started to kick in, so he

lay down on the sofa for a short doze.
Next thing he knew, the room was full of
smoke, there's banging on the door, sirens
out in the street. Now he was in A&E for
the effects of smoke inhalation.

A&E Registrar, Derby

Read the Label

A colleague of mine took a call from a patient who'd been prescribed antibiotics. The patient had a recurrent infection, and as such his GP felt he warranted a ten-day course to be sure of clearing the infection this time.

The GP had asked him to take his antibiotics four times daily for ten days. Three days later he called NHS Direct, in obvious distress, to ask if he really needed the full course, as they were making him feel really weak. This was not a side effect anyone would expect, so my colleague asked him what made him think it was the medication doing this.

'Well,' he said, 'I'm sure the doctor said the tablets are to be taken on an empty stomach so I have had nothing to eat for three days…'

GP, NHS Direct

Diminished Responsibility

We're taking a lovely young woman to hospital following an attempted suicide, when she says, 'Do you know the great thing about hearing voices?'

'You hear voices?' I asked.

'Yes. I do. I hear voices…' she wiggles her bandaged right hand in the air above her head. 'And they tell me to do all kinds of mad things. Cut your arm, Sarah. Stab that dog, Sarah. Sarah, swear at those people. But…' she leans forward, conspiratorially, '…the great thing is: *I'm not responsible.*'

Community Psychiatric Nurse, Chester

Thong Place at the Thong Time

One of my colleagues told me about a man they were called out to on an early, rather chilly, November morning. He was called Tam, and was adamant that he was fine.

He told them he'd had a wee tumble down an embankment and been halted by a no parking sign. He was covered in scratches and was wearing nothing but a thong, which immediately got alarm bells ringing.

She asked him not to move whilst they checked him over, and while they were doing that she asked him what had happened. He said he was walking along the top of the embankment when two youths accosted him and demanded he take some Viagra, and when he'd politely declined they shoved him down the slope. The following exchange then took place:

Medic: But why are you only dressed in a thong, Tam?

Patient: Well, I imagine my clothes were ripped from me as I hurtled down the slope.

[At this moment a member of the public

*brings over a bag of clothes found in
the bushes]*

   Medic: Are these yours?

   Patient: Yes! Oh, how wonderful of you!

   Medic: But you said they'd been torn off?

   Patient: Well, obviously that kind person
must have collected them for me - how nice!

Paramedic, Glasgow

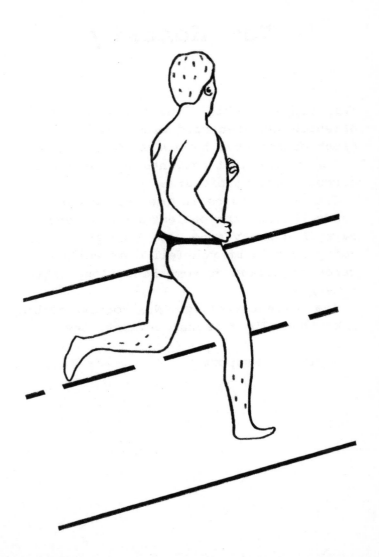

Raw Honesty

This happened when I was training, part of which involved shadowing a particularly blunt doctor when he was on duty in A&E.

One of the last patients we see has a carrot stuck up his arse.

The doctor comes in (me following), reads through the patient's notes, and says in a weary tone, 'So I suppose you're going to tell me you fell over whilst gardening naked or something along those lines, eh?'

The patient replies, 'No, doctor, nothing like that. I'm a sexual deviant, see.'

Consultant, Newport

Taxi-ing Situation

A young woman thinks she may have broken her ankle, so she dials the number of her local taxi firm. The taxi arrives, and she get in gingerly, saying, 'To the hospital please, I think I've broken my ankle.' The taxi driver takes umbrage at this, whips out his phone and dials 999. My colleague gets the call. She asks him to drive the woman to hospital, which he refuses, shouting that the woman is entitled to an ambulance. My colleague says that she'd love to send an ambulance, but that it would be safer for the woman if she was just driven there in the vehicle she is currently in.

'Is that right, mate?' says the taxi driver, and hangs up. A few minutes later he calls again. In a triumphant voice he says, 'We've got her out! Now, send an ambulance.' And hangs up again.

To be fair to the man, he did stay with her until the ambulance arrived, if only to shout at them for not doing their duty.

Call handler, Croydon

Bobby Dangler

We admitted a red-faced sixteen-year-old male who was covered in piercings. He was in because, in a friend's shed, he'd DIYed a piercing to his frenulum (a bit of skin just beneath the glans of the penis) and – surprise, surprise – it was infected. His mother had brought him in, and kept saying, 'I told you, no more bloody piercings, what did I tell you?'

I was impressed that he'd done it without anaesthetic.

Nurse, Norwich

Out on a Limb

I was called out on the bike to a man who had been trying to saw a branch off a tree in his garden with a handsaw, unsurprisingly with limited success. Once he'd got through halfway, and was very much out of breath, he decided the best thing would be to loop a rope around the bough, and see if he could tug it off. So he got his son to climb up the tree and tie a rope where he'd been cutting, and then started to heave at it. According to the son, the branch wasn't giving in that easily, so the father had to really put his back into it. Then eventually, with an almighty crack, he succeeded, and the whole tree came straight down. On top of him, that is. Luckily, his wife's ornamental fountain slowed it just enough that he didn't get completely flattened, but he did have several broken bones.

First Responder Paramedic, London

Devil Finds Work for Idle Hands

A muppet presents to hospital with a broken ankle. Apparently he'd had the brilliant idea of strapping a windsurfing sail to a homemade skateboard, then took it to a car park in 20 knot winds, realised he was going too fast and was running out of car park, so stepped off. Crack.

Apparently the first time he had tried (yes, there was more than one attempt), there was only a very gentle breeze, and he was convinced he was a genius.

The age of this 'genius'? 35. Thirty five years of age. Windsurfing with a skateboard.

We made sure he told everyone working that shift his sorry tale.

Orthopaedic Registrar, Plymouth

Pants on Fire

In the days of house visits I attended a guy who had managed to get an orange lodged firmly inside his rectal cavity. Perhaps suprisingly, a not uncommon occurrence. When I went into the house, he was waddling around in a pair of tiny denim shorts, and no top.

I asked him what happened. He said he had been painting the ceiling when he lost his footing and fell onto the fruit bowl. Now, under certain circumstances (i.e. a fruit with a more invasive shape), this could be a physically possible if implausible excuse. However, there wasn't a ladder or paintbrush in sight…

It would be a difficult extraction. At one point, to my shame, my professionalism slipped and I suggested banging him against a table top like a Terry's Chocolate Orange to see if the segments would come out individually.

GP, Norwich

Put a Sock in It

In the mid-90s I was helping out in A&E on a busy Saturday night. A guy was brought in from an unofficial rave by ambulance, after having apparently danced so much he passed out. We suspected a Class A drugs overdose. When he came in, he was wearing an extremely tight pair of white jeans, and he had an astonishingly large bulge down one leg. The trousers were so tight that they had to be cut off him (he was still unconscious at this point, and we wanted to insert a catheter, honest). After cutting them off, fully anticipating something prodigious, we were disappointed to discover what the huge bulge really was - a football sock stuffed with cotton wool.

Nurse, Dundee

No Eye Dear

I work as a specialist nurse in a care home. An elderly lady was in clinic, and I asked her if she could read the eye chart for me, covering her left eye.

Patient: I can't, dear.

Me: Ok, cover your other eye and read the chart.

Patient: I still can't I'm afraid, dear.

Me: (thinking for a moment) Can you read, Rosie?

Patient: Of course I can, dear!

Me: But you can't read the chart?

Patient: No.

Me: Can you *see* the chart (I was getting slightly irritable by this stage)?

Patient: Oh, yes, dearie.

Me: Then why can't you read it?

Patient: Because I can't pronounce it!

Nurse, Welwyn Garden City

Ship of Fools

When I was training, a group of medical students I knew went out on a stag night, got the groom very drunk, and when they got back to his flat decided to catheterise him and fill the balloon (which lies in the bladder to keep the tube in place) with plaster of paris. The result? The wedding had to be replaced with a very painful operation. Though one of my old friends, who was a ringleader, still has the plaster mould in his possession. I like to think that the bride-to-be threw it at him.

Consultant Anaesthetist, Durham

Bathing Beauty

Our former district nurse, back in the days when patients were still given baths, was asked to visit a lady who she had not met before.

The unkempt patient answered the door, seemed a little younger than the nurse had imagined and rather confused about the appointment, but appeared grateful to be getting a wash. The nurse assumed she was an early-onset dementia sufferer.

She gave the rather grubby lady a lovely bath and washed her hair. The patient was overjoyed with the experience, and arranged for the nurse to come back the following week for the same again.

On returning to the clinic, the Sister in charge asked her why she hadn't visited the old lady that day. Of course, it turned out the nurse had bathed the patient's neighbour!

Practice Nurse, Ashton-under-Lyme

Tick Tock, Up My Cock

As a medical student, I once saw an X-ray showing a rather large watch (I never found out what make) sitting low in a patient's bladder. Shocked, I asked the consultant how it could have got there – surely the urethra is too small. The consultant looked at me, back at the X-ray and shrugged, saying, 'In my profession, you quickly find out that if someone wants a certain object in a certain orifice, they will make it so.'

Since that day, I have found that to be the case. Although there are limits and perversion is constrained to an extent by orifice diameter.

Saying that, I later found out I had been victim of a common rite-of-passage wheeze where a watch is taped inside the waistband of the patient's underpants before the X-ray.

A&E Consultant, Manchester

Shedding Light on the Matter

As a new student, I had a placement in A&E – this was in Blackpool, which, being a party town, was quite scary, with lots of drunks etc. I was asked to monitor a patient for neurological observations following a fall. The gentle man was rather dishevelled and stank of alcohol, and I was new to the job and petrified!

Part of my monitoring included checking blood pressure, reflexes and pupil dilation. I was extremely worried that one eye reacted normally to my pen torch but the other didn't, so I called for help and in stepped a consultant. He had been leading some other students around, so they gathered round also, to my great embarrassment.

After a short examination, the consultant stood back, and with a completely straight face announced that the lack of movement was due to the patient being the proud owner of a glass eye!

GP, Lancaster

Still Life

When I was Sister on the Oncology ward we once had an old man die after quite some time in hospital, just before visiting time. I asked a couple of student nurses to prepare the body for the family, in other words make him look as natural as possible to minimise their distress.

When they finished they came and told me they felt they'd managed to get him as natural as they could. I went in to his room to check they had done everything correctly. I was astonished to see the old man sat on the bed, legs crossed, dressed in his pyjamas, slippers and dressing gown, with a newspaper propped on his chest open at the crossword, and a pen clutched in his hand.

Ward Sister, London

Blown it

A man came in with his penis caught in his fly – apparently his girlfriend had given him a blowjob, and then decided to do him up with her teeth – not the most accurate of instruments for that task. We got it out with pliers and only minimal foreskin chafing – interesting marks that looked like he'd been gnawed by a pair of hungry gerbils.

A&E Registrar, Falkirk

Fist Aid

For some reason people never understand why the presence of a first aider at the scene of an accident only makes us drive faster. Here's why:

We were called to a restaurant where a man had suffered a suspected heart attack. The notes stated that there was a 'first aider on scene'.

When we arrived we found the patient fully conscious, but with a huge amount of chest pain. It turns out that when the customer fainted, a customer on the other side of the restaurant jumped up, shouted, 'Don't worry, I'm a trained first aider,' and before even checking for vital signs started on CPR.

Whilst he's thumping away with his fist, the patient wakes up and starts screaming, though the first aider doesn't stop, just keeps shouting 'It's all right, mate, I'm a trained first aider!' until staff manage to pull him off.

The hapless diner ended up having to

spend a night in hospital with three
broken ribs. The first aider had vanished,
without even paying for his meal.

Paramedic, Dover

Meat is Murder

A woman came to the surgery during the height of the swine flu panic. I diagnosed her with a mild case of the illness, sent off some tests and told her to go home, rest and take regular fluids and paracetamol.

She looked at me, incredulous and angry. 'That's impossible,' she said. It can't be swine flu. I'm a strict vegetarian.'

GP, London

Suffer a Jet

I once treated a healthy young woman who presented with acute onset of abdominal pain and found her to have extensive pneumoperitoneum – which means she had air in her abdomen.

And where did the air come from? It was 'Jacuzzi-jet-induced' she admitted.

Consultant Surgeon, Harrogate

Anatomy Lessons

A 19-year-old female came into A&E and I asked her what the problem was. She said that she and her boyfriend were having sex and the condom came off and she wasn't able to retrieve it with her fingers. She then went to the bathroom and stuck two fingers down her throat, but apparently she couldn't vomit it up either…

Triage Nurse, Slough

Nailed

Working on the call desk of the Glaswegian ambulance service, I got this call from, shall we say, a rather rough area.

'Alright, pal, I need to get someone to have a look at my leg.'

'OK, what is the matter with it?'

'Ah wiz takin a telly oot a flat on Wednesday, right, when ah saw the polis drive up the road, but, so ah thought to mesel, Ahm nae gonna get lifted for this, eh, cause ah'm on bail, ken, so ah dropped it and jumped o'er a coupla fences and made aff. Problem is, ah didnae see this nail, right, and it did mah leg…'

'I see, so you'd like me to get you an ambulance for a cut to the leg you sustained yesterday, whilst running from the police?'

'Aye, that's right, hen, so send me the fuckin ambulance, now!'

It wasn't an ambulance I sent to that address that night.

Call handler, Glasgow

Blade Runner

A teenager was brought in with concussion and a small cut on his forehead, which had been bleeding profusely. It was only superficial, however, and didn't need stitching. When we asked him how it had happened, he went bright red, and very quietly said he'd been shaving in the shower and had fallen over. Puzzled, I mentioned that that didn't sound very embarrassing, to which he replied, 'Um, I wasn't shaving *up there*, I was shaving *downstairs*.'

Nurse, Wrexham